My Dad Naps Too!

Part of the Talking to Kids About Narcolepsy Series

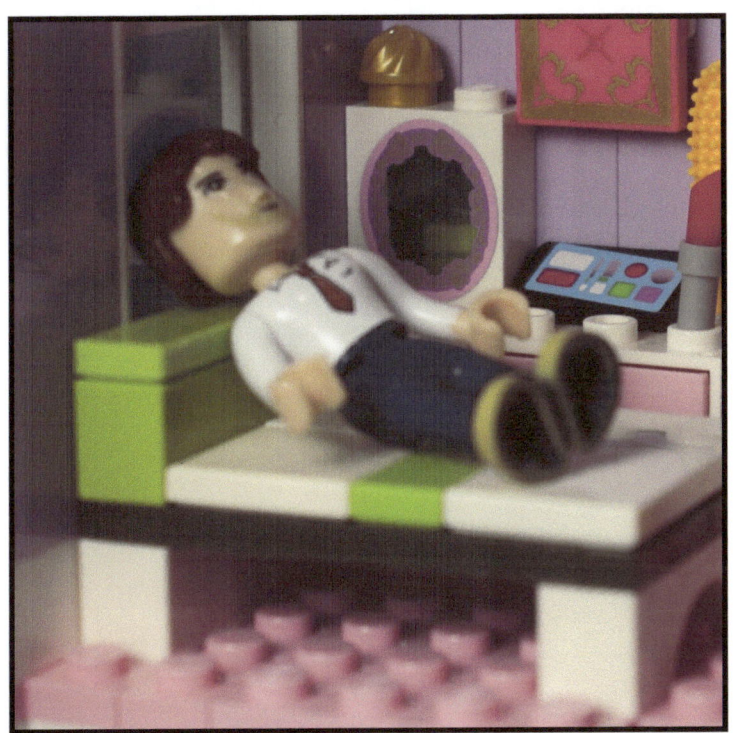

A Book About Narcolepsy and Excessive Daytime Sleepiness

To my Grampy,

Your kindness and love have always helped me find my way

To my Dad,

It took 30 years for us to find each other, I am so happy to have that missing piece in my life at last.

My Dad Naps Too!

A Book About Narcolepsy and Excessive Daytime Sleepiness

Amanda Stock

astock204@gmail.com

ISBN-13: 978-1516888191

ISBN-10: 151688197

First Edition 2015

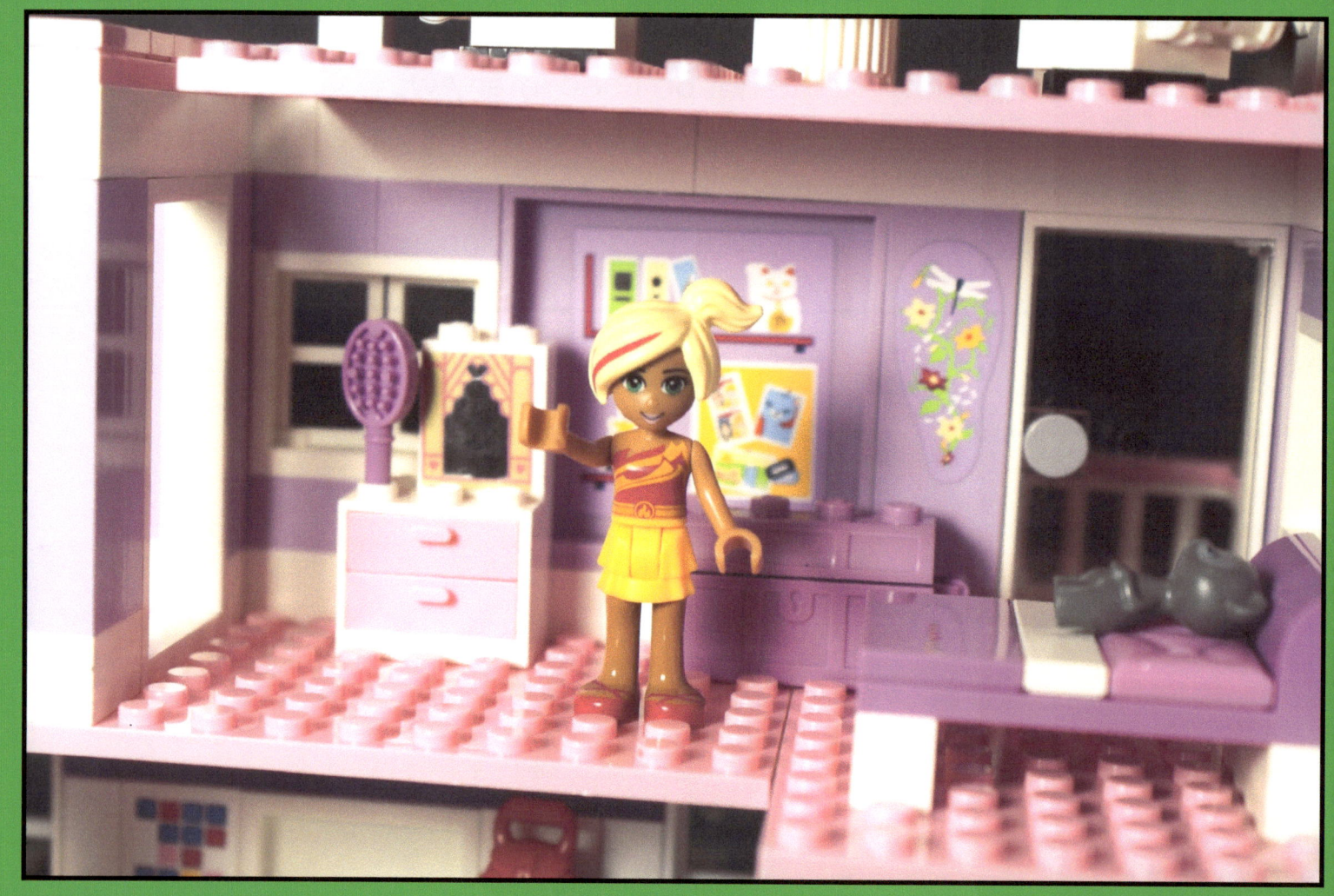

Hi! My name is Jennifer.

My dad is the best science teacher in the whole world! He gets up early to be at school before his students but when he comes home from school he is so tired he has to take a nap.

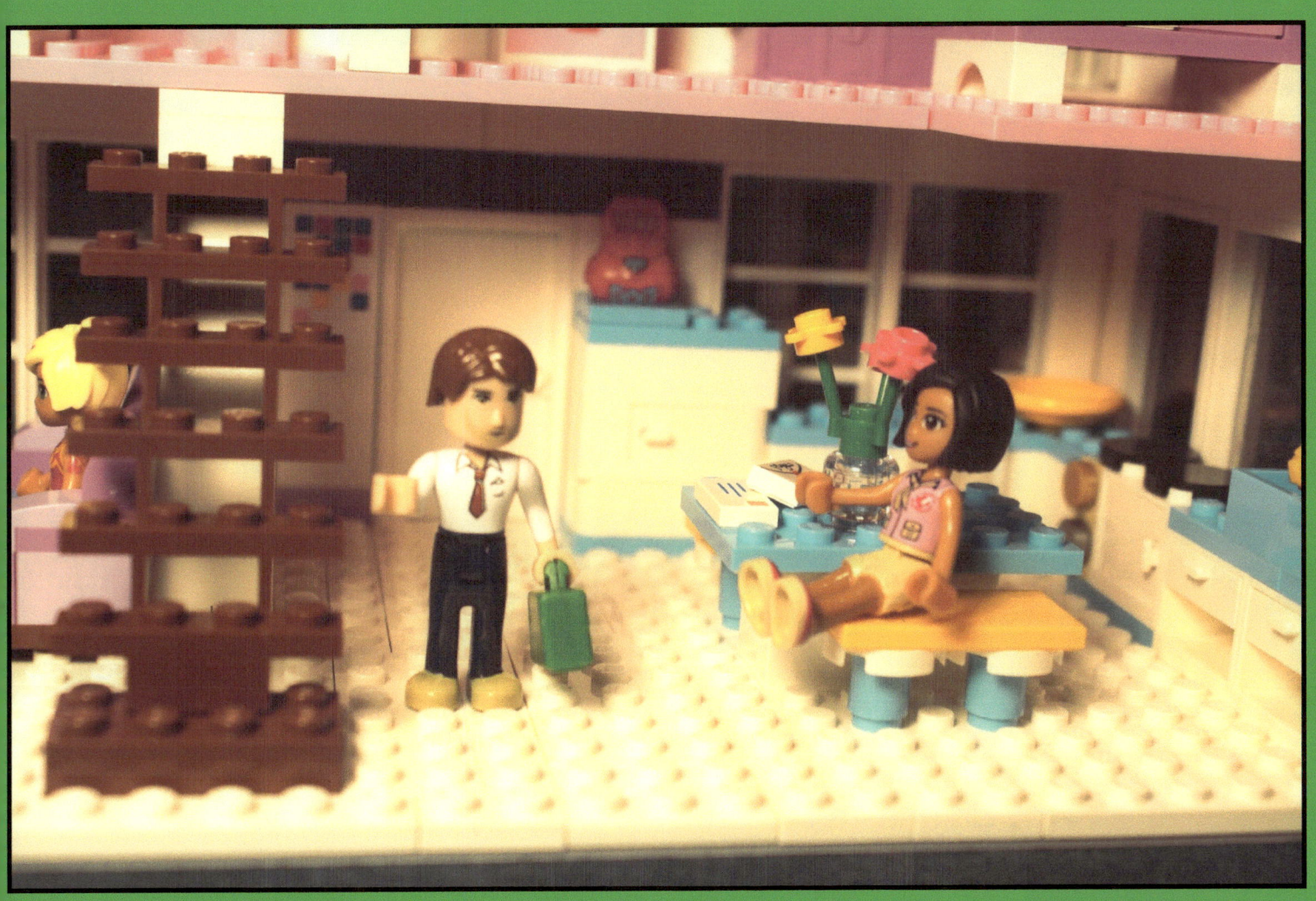

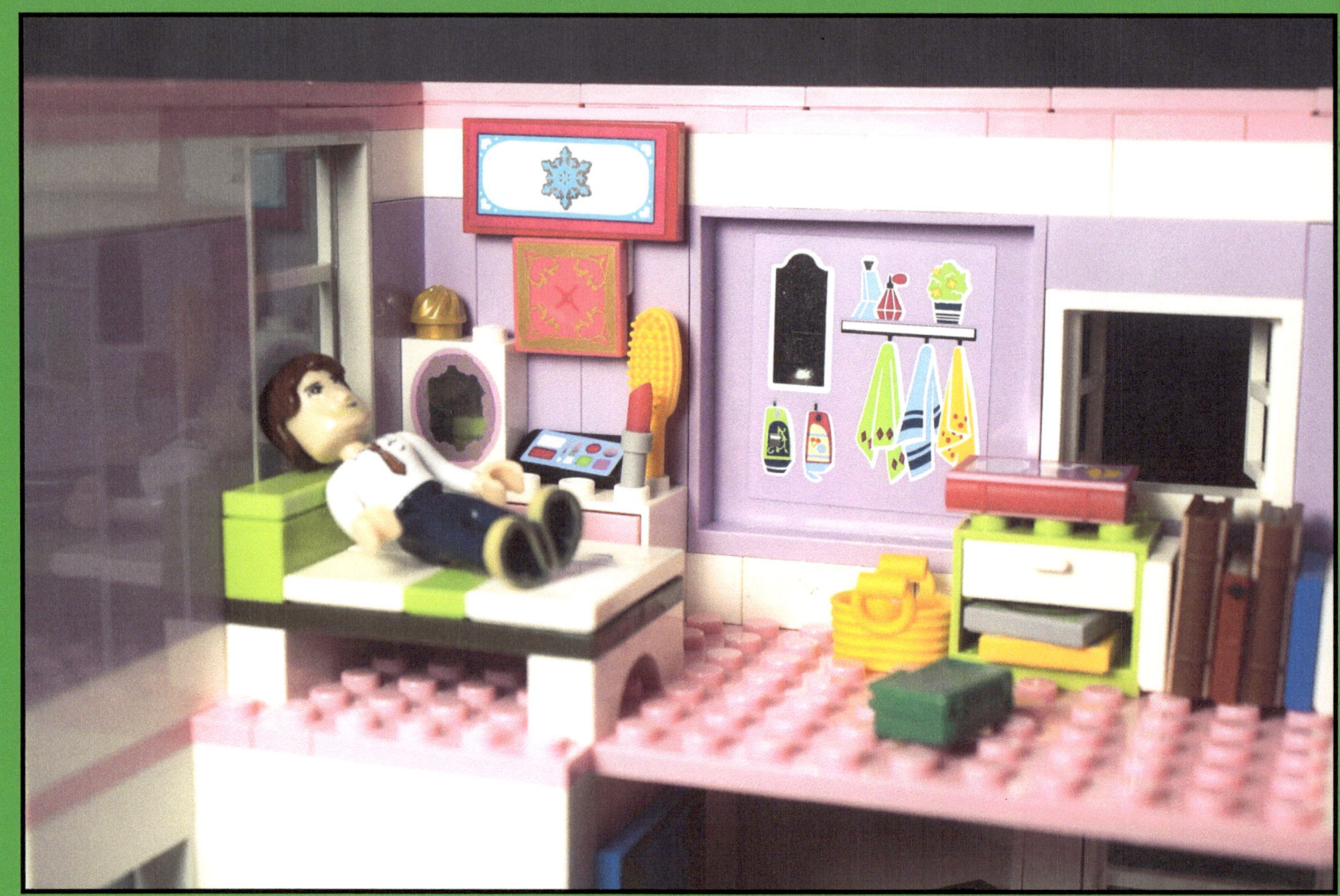

I used to think that only babies needed naps so I asked my mom. She told me dad has a sleep disorder called Narcolepsy.

Narcolepsy makes my daddy sleepy all the time because his brain keeps him up at night and doesn't tell him to stay awake during the day the way mine does. When I go to sleep I sleep all night and wake up feeling great!

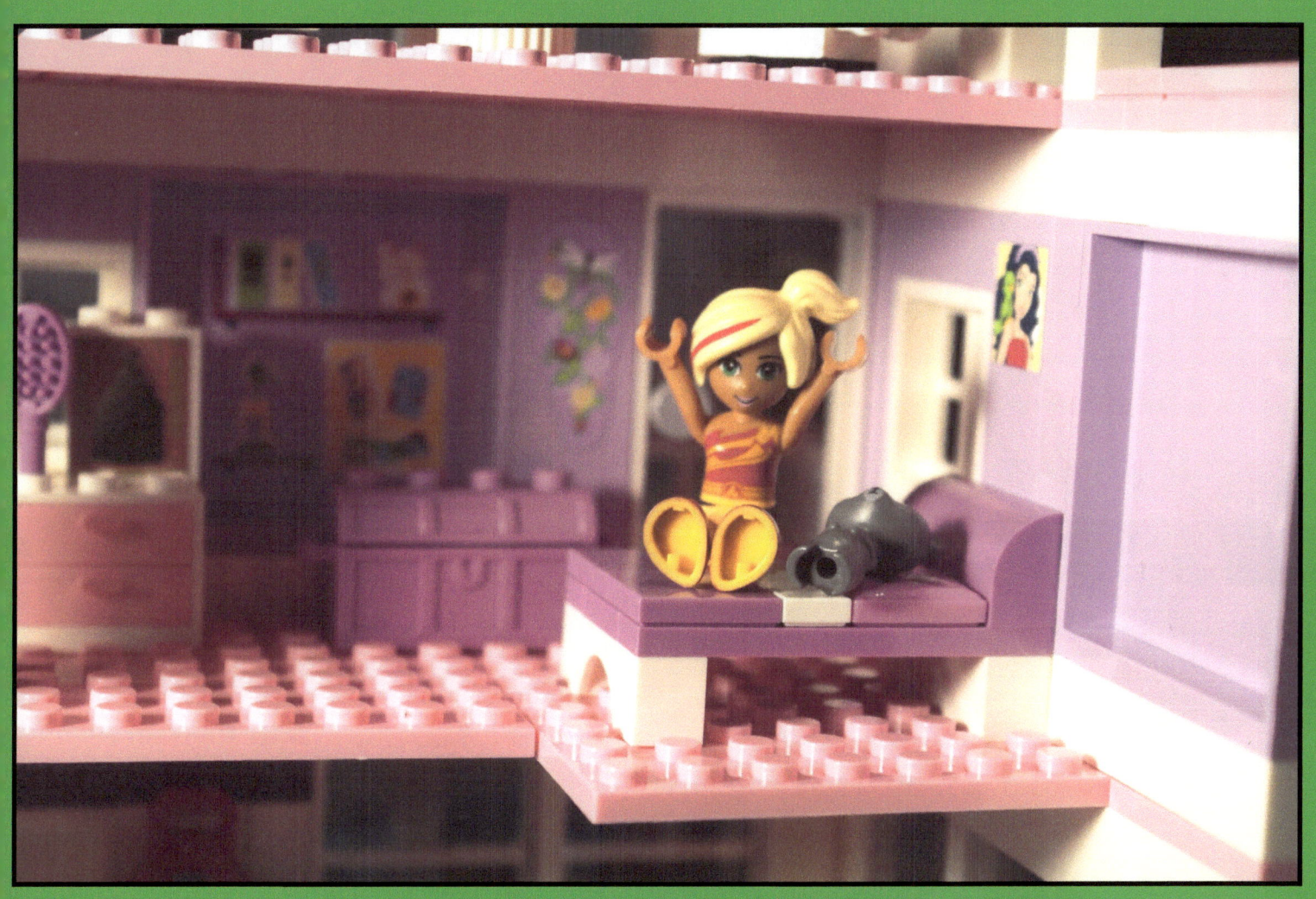

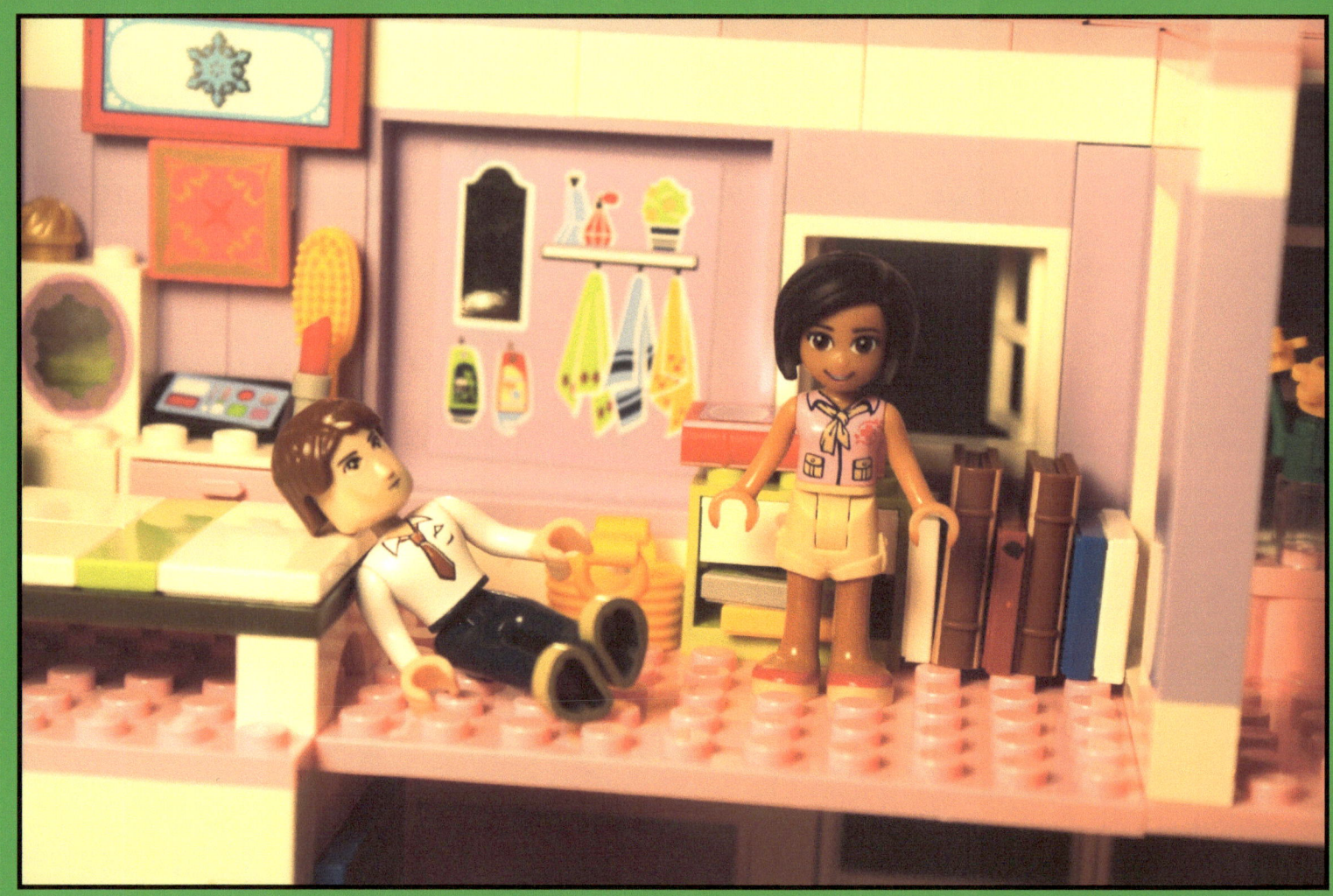

When my daddy goes to sleep he wakes up a lot at night and he still feels sleepy in the morning. Mommy says he has a symptom of Narcolepsy called Excessive Daytime Sleepiness.

Excessive Daytime Sleepiness makes going to work hard for him. Sometimes dad gets so tired he has to sit down and he falls asleep, even when he is in the middle of teaching.

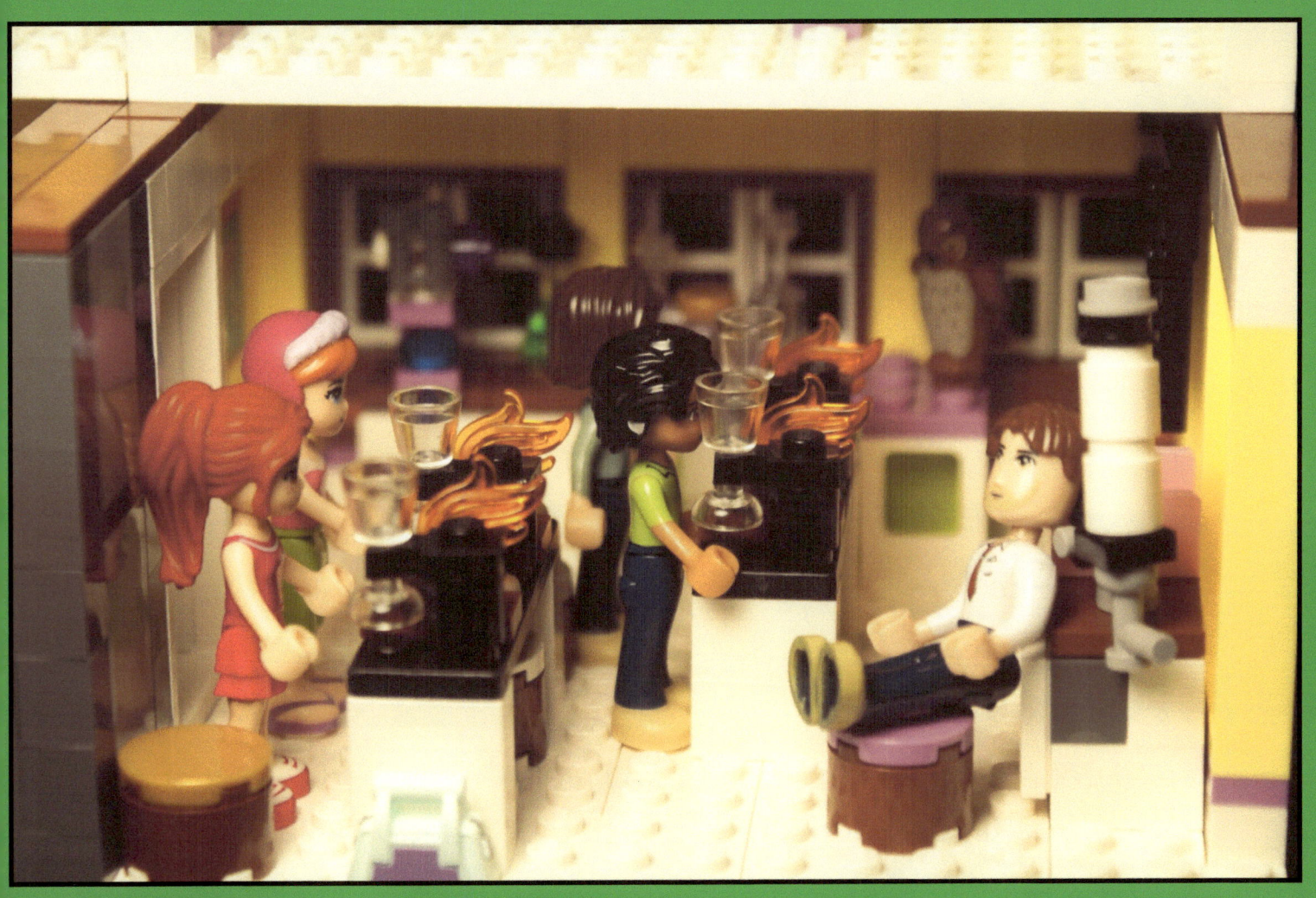

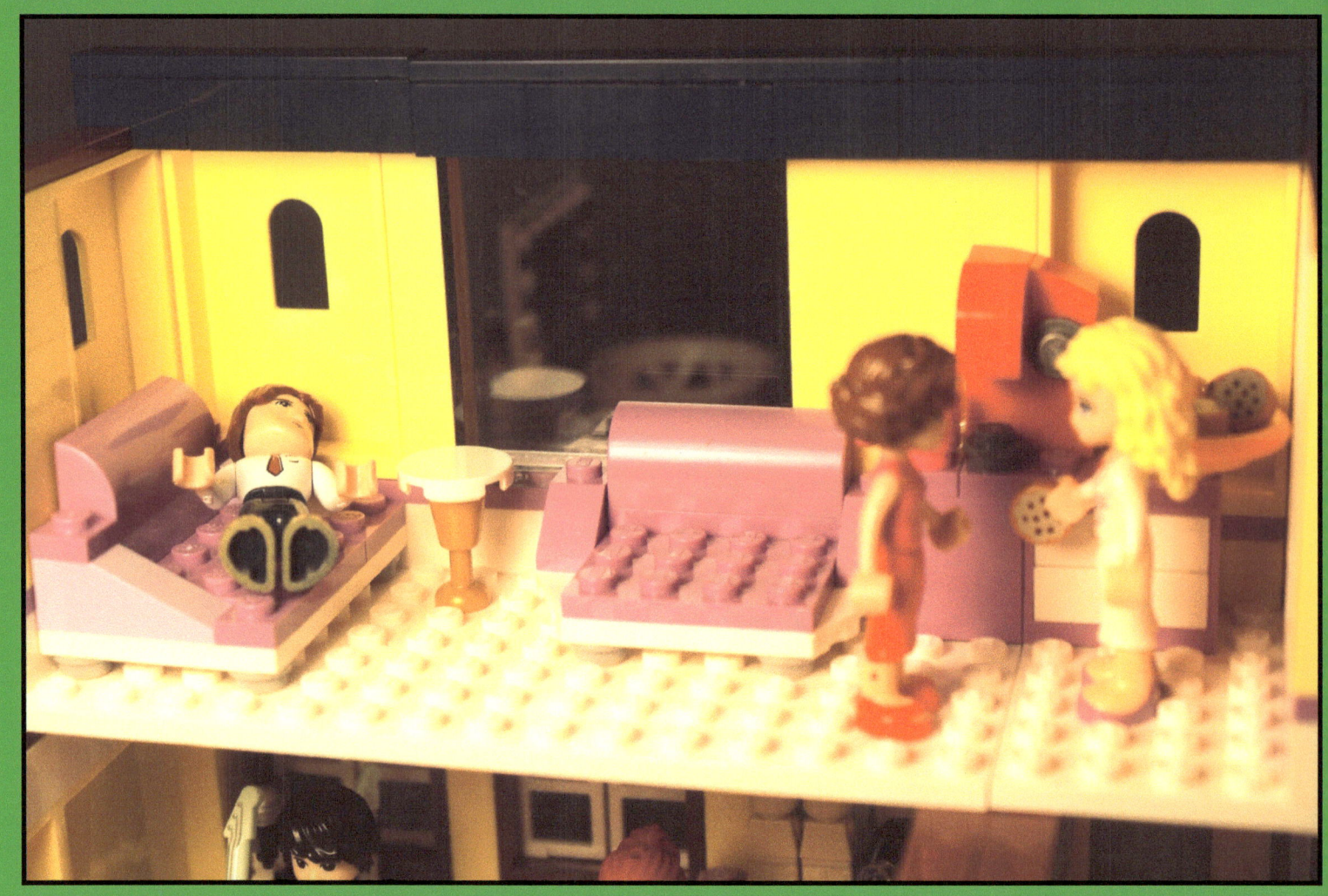

He had to get a note from his doctor saying he is allowed to nap during his free time at work so he doesn't fall asleep in class.

Teachers need to stand all day and that takes a lot of energy. Dad needs to walk around and make sure everyone is doing their science projects safely. Narcolepsy can make it very hard to concentrate That can get dangerous but as long has he follows his doctor's instructions he is ok to go to work every day.

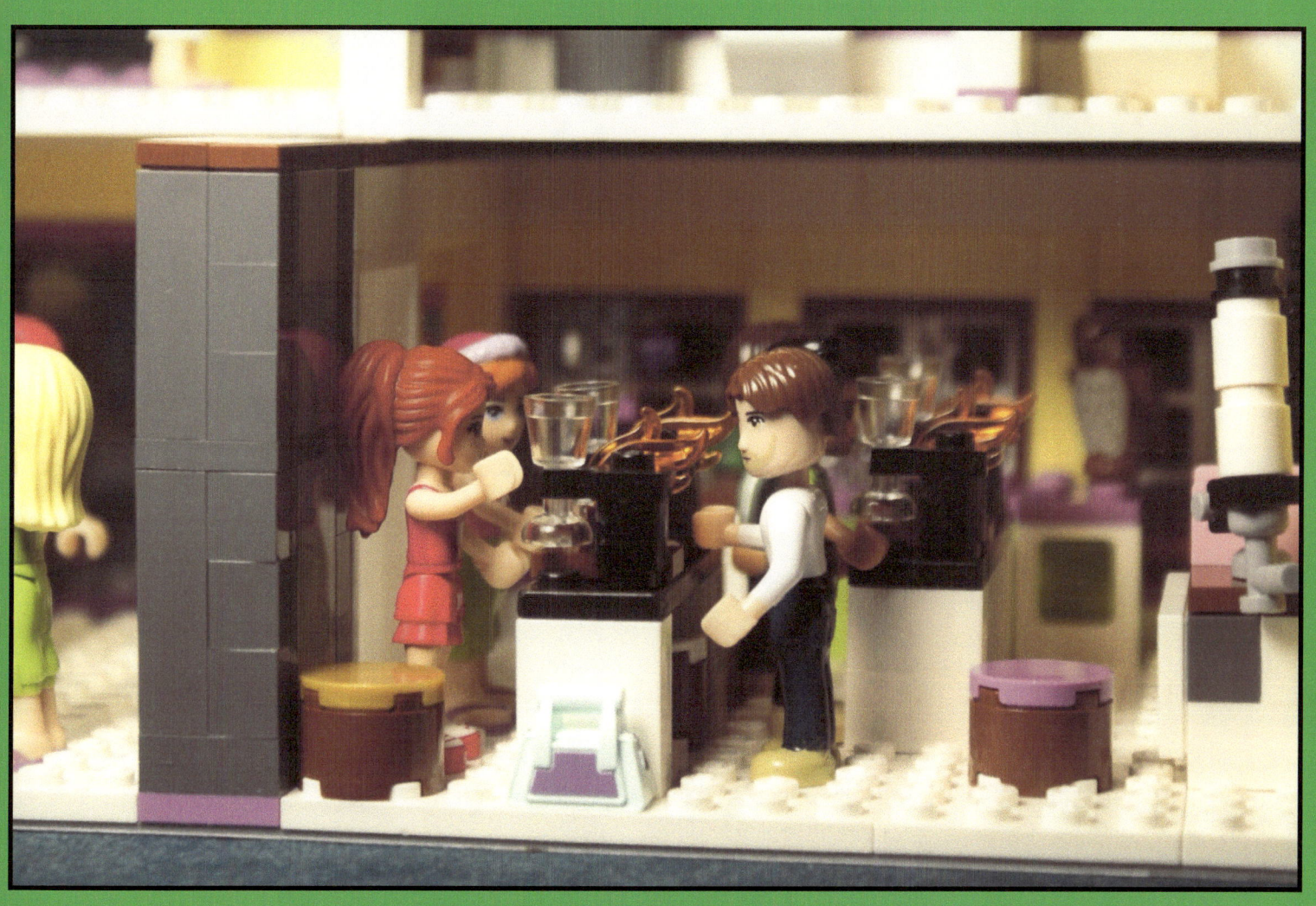

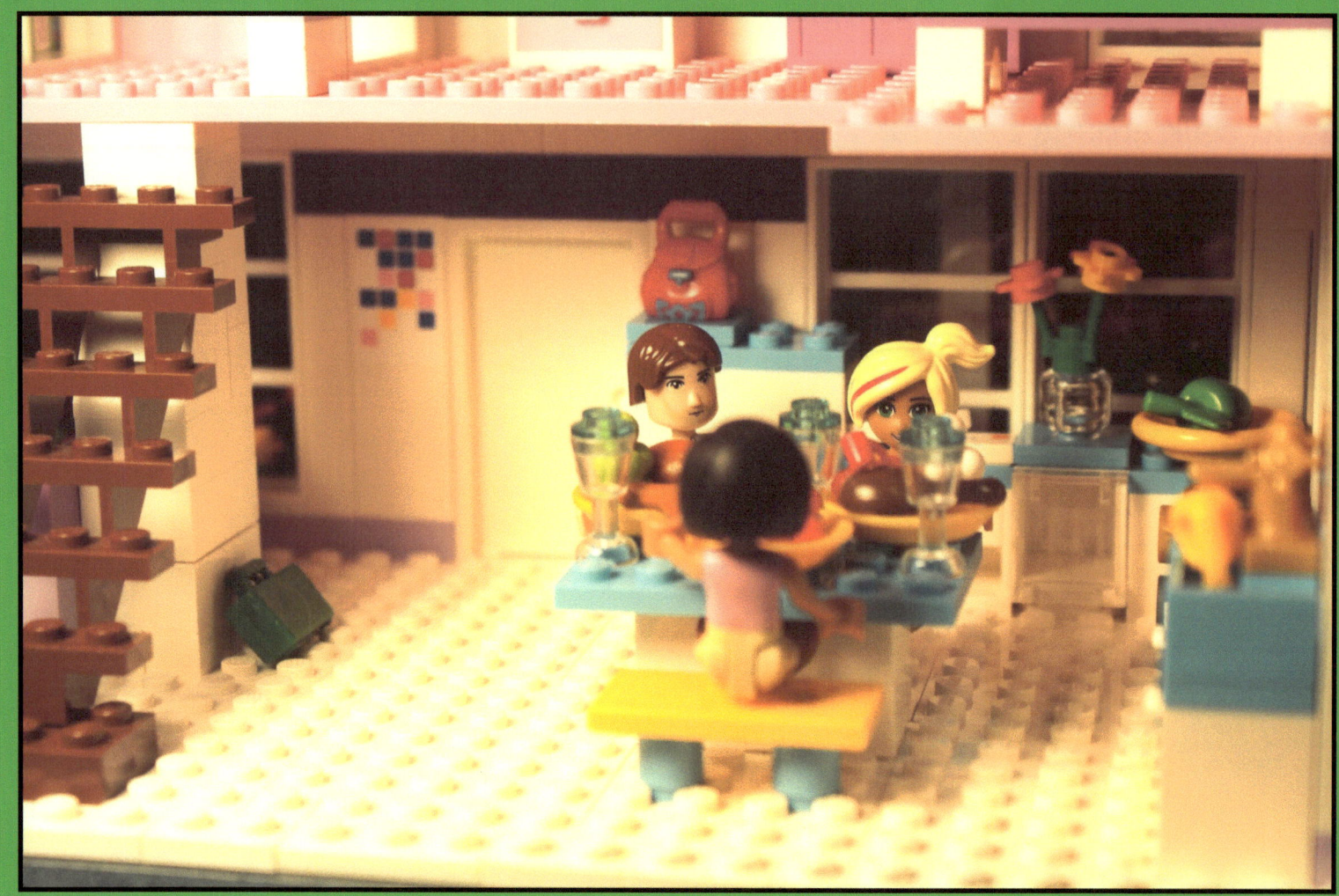

Dad takes special medication to keep the Narcolepsy away. As a family we eat healthy foods and dad exercises when he has the energy, but being a teacher has long hours and he doesn't get to exercise as much as he would like.

He also has a bed time just like me. He told me keeping a sleep schedule helps him feel better.

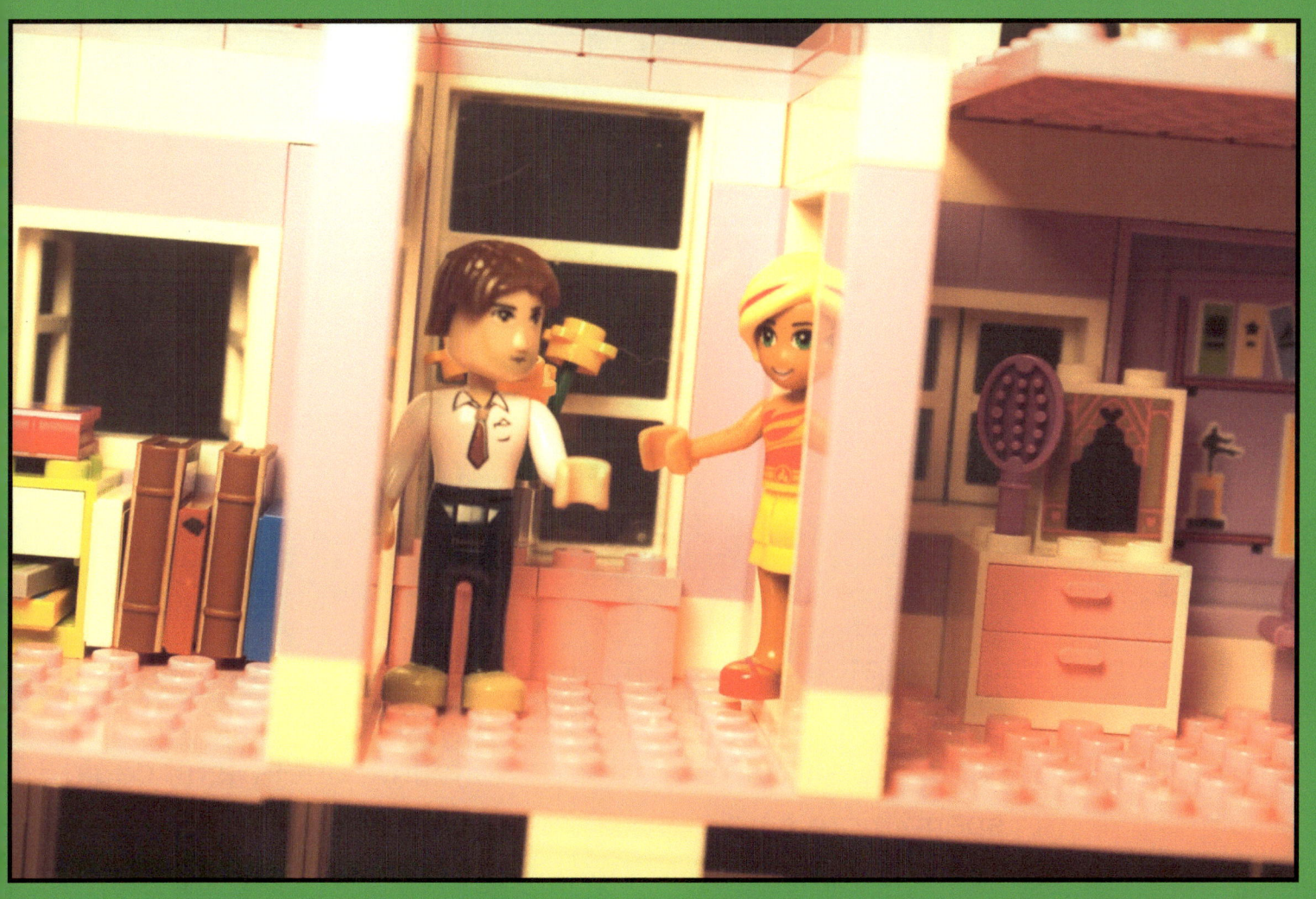

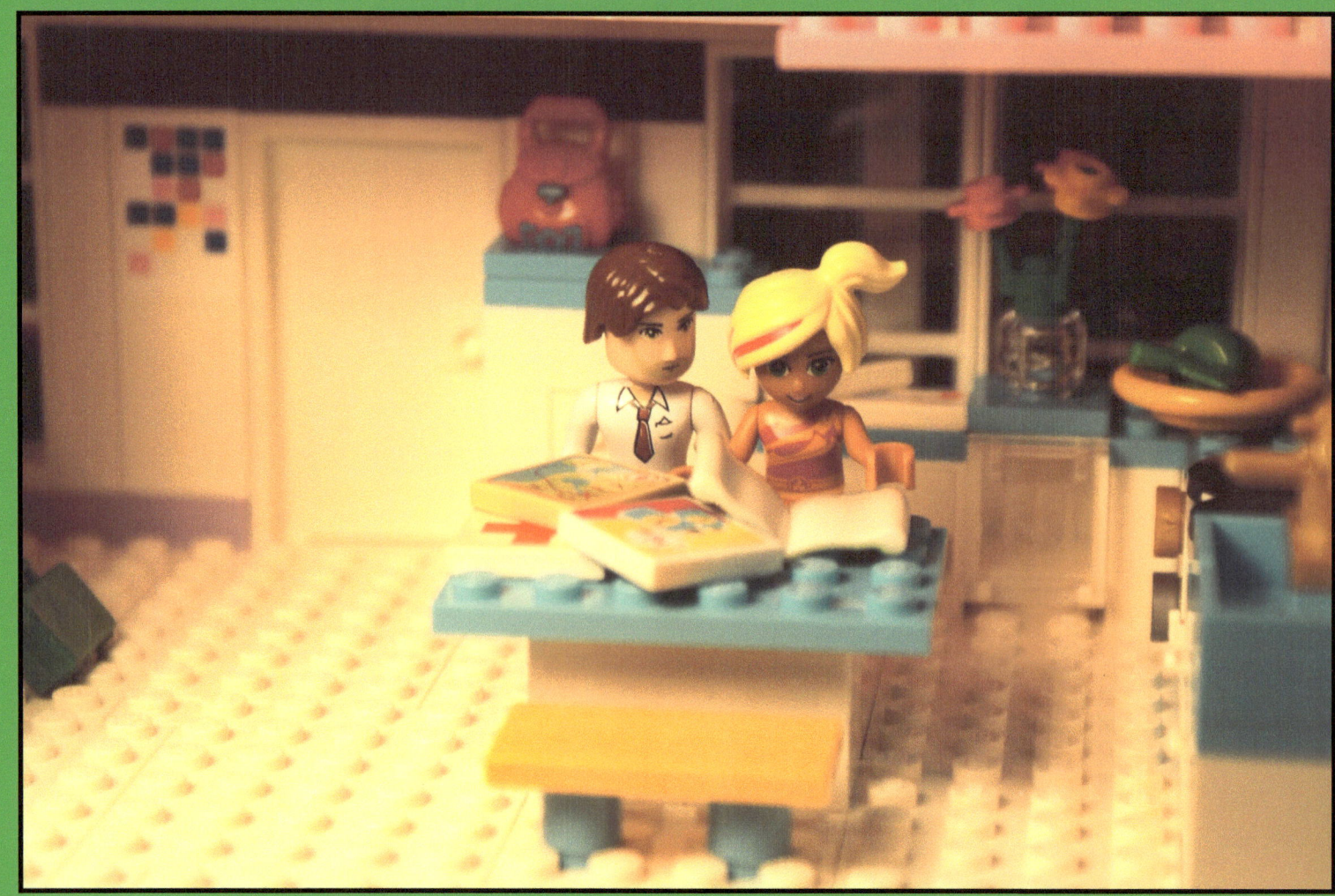

When he takes naps after school it means that I do not get to see him until dinner time. If he does not have papers to grade he helps me with my homework after we eat. I like our homework time but I wish I could spend more time with him on school days.

Sometimes Dad has to stay up late to grade papers and not sleeping makes him very cranky. When he is tired sometimes he yells and is mean so I hide until he feels better.

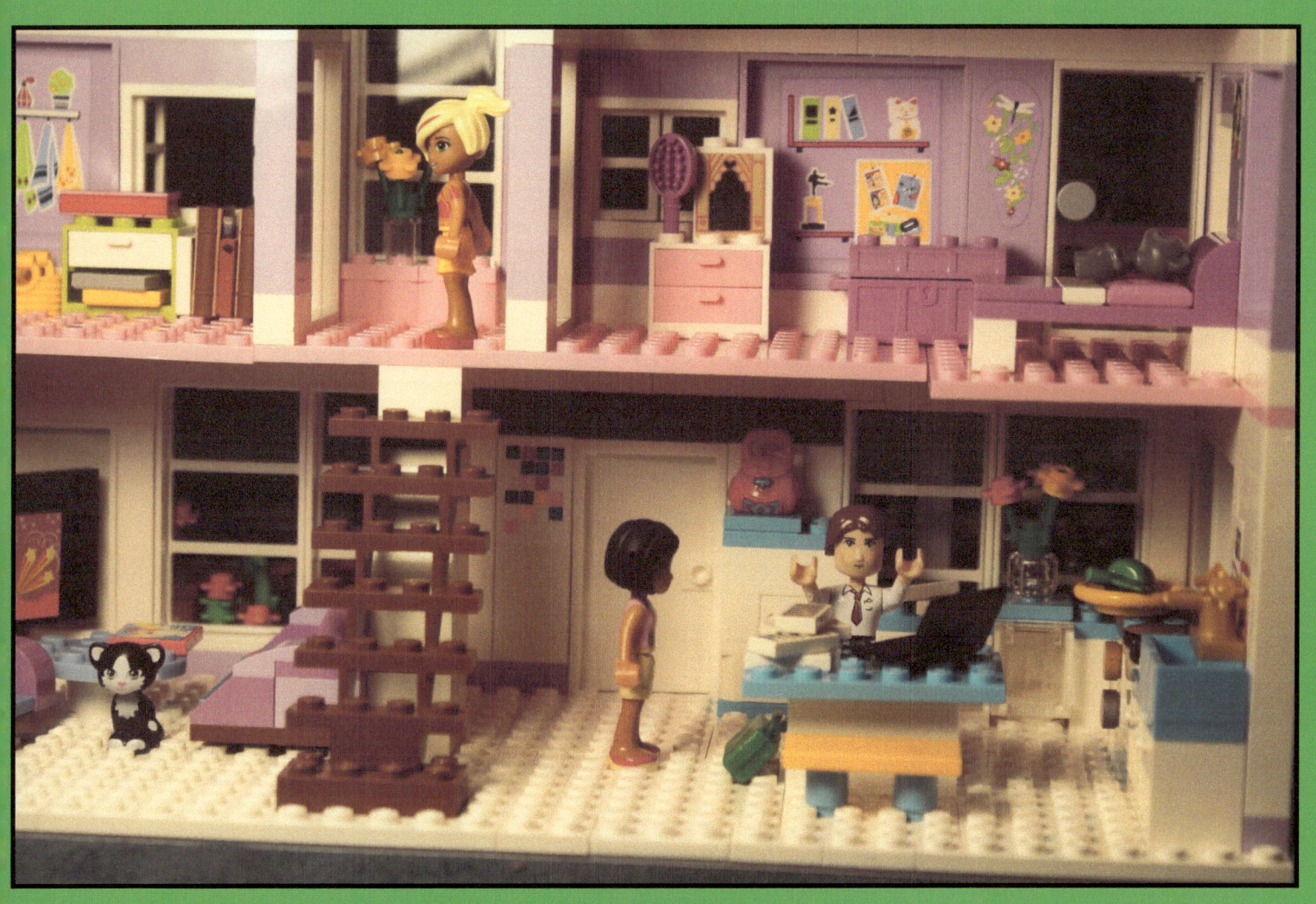

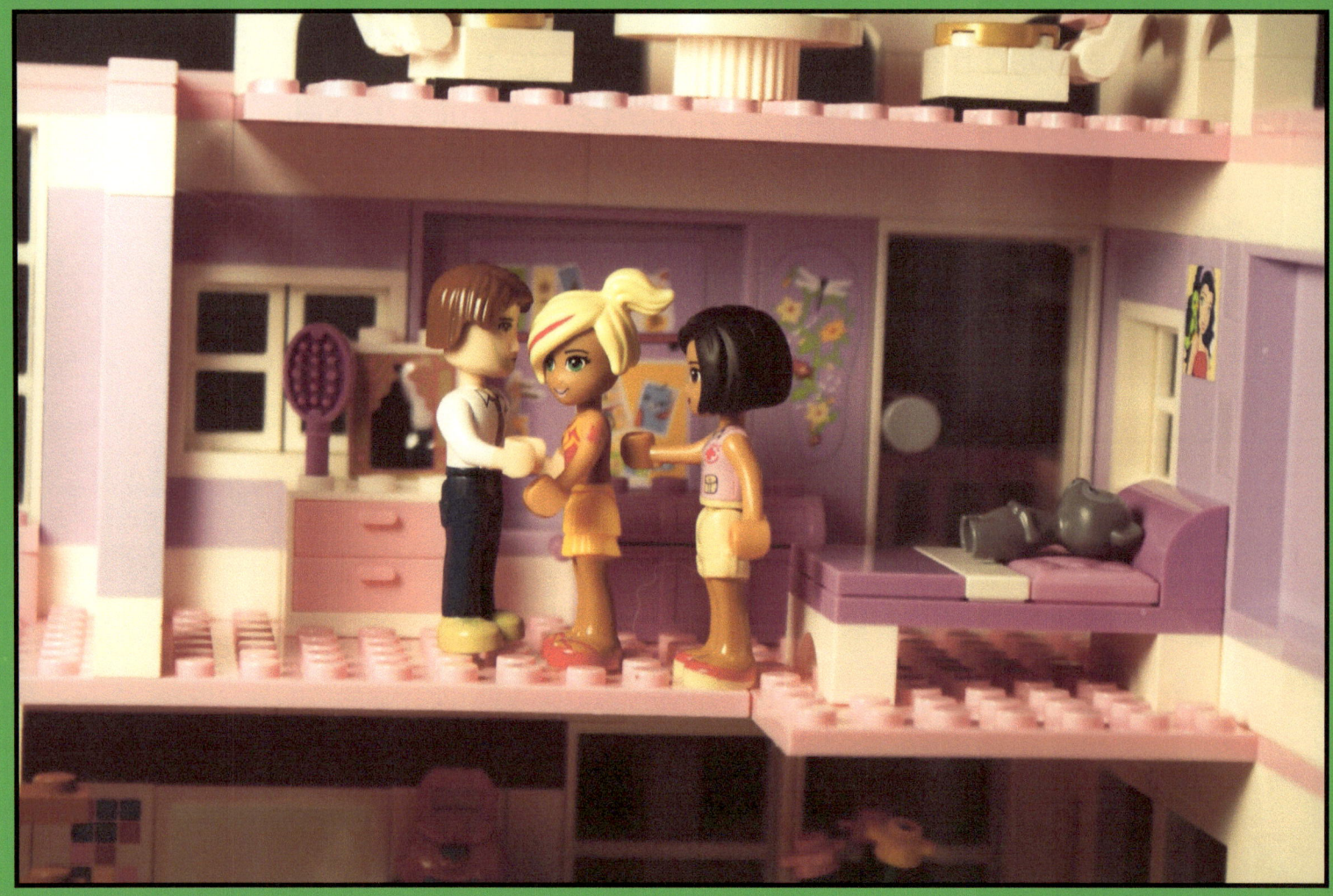

Mom told me that dad hates how Narcolepsy can make him act and he does not like himself when he is tired. He loves me and never wants to be the reason why I am sad.

Dad can drive when he takes his medication and naps. Sometimes he gets a ride with another teacher in the mornings and mom picks him up when school is done.

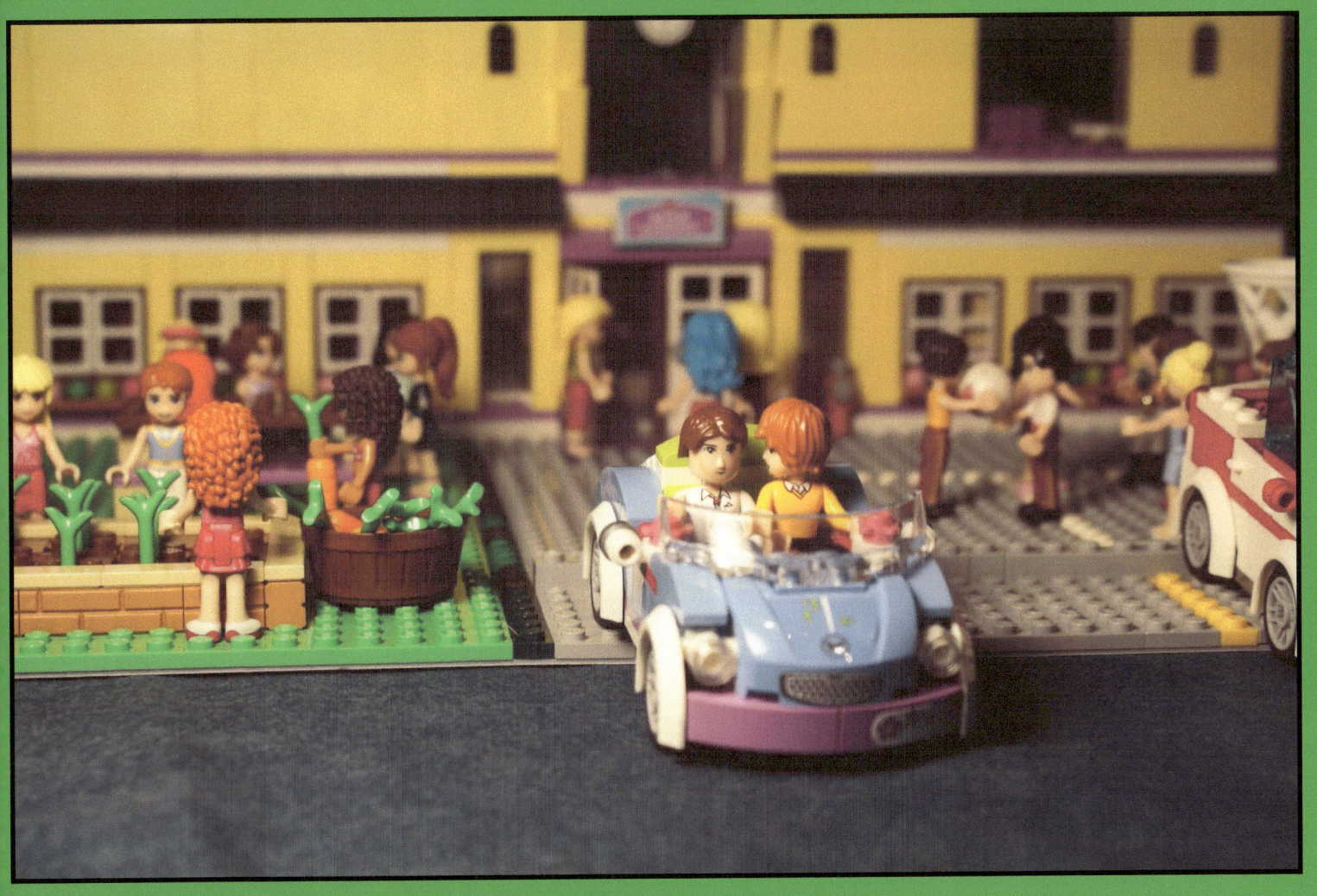

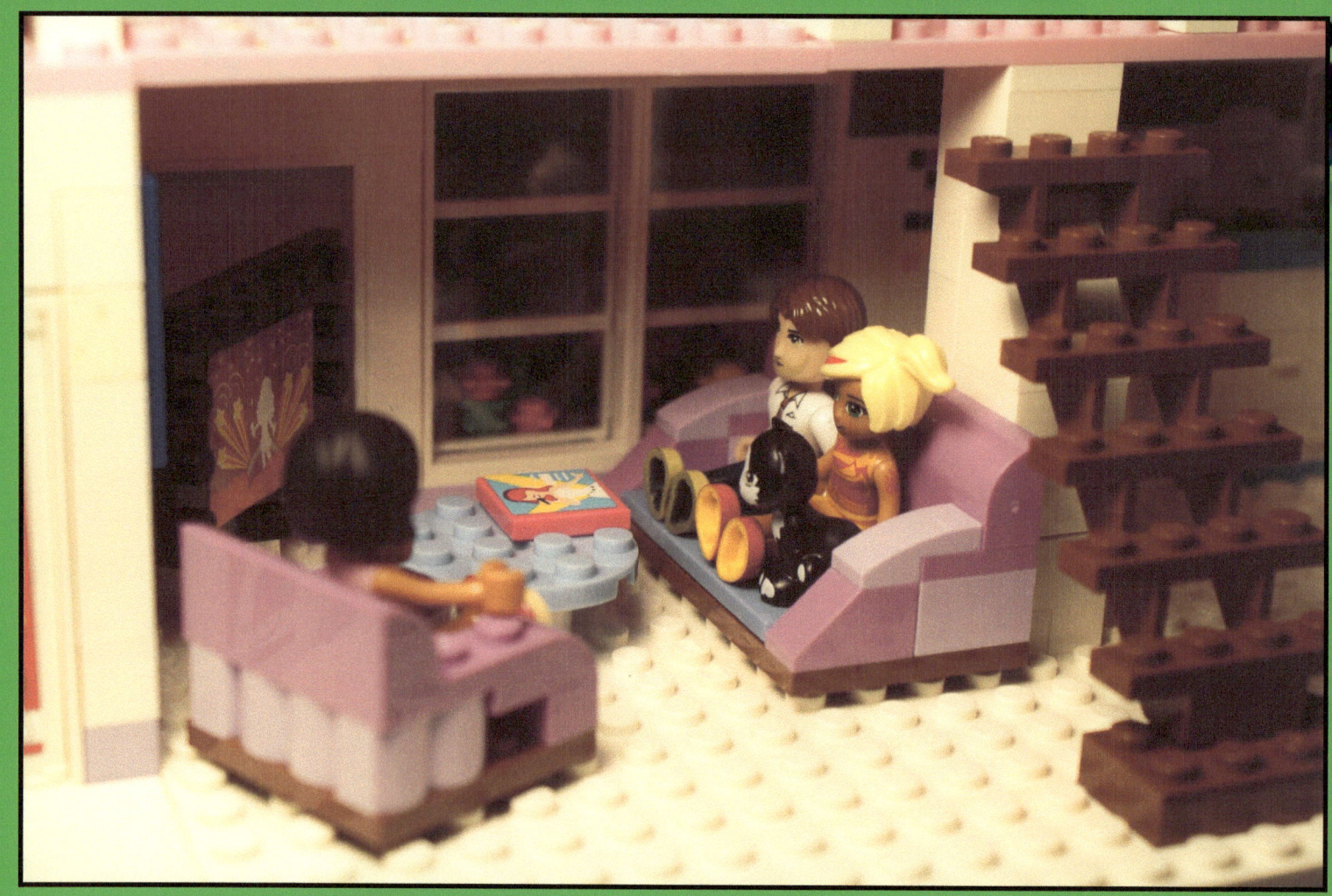

Living with Narcolepsy can be really hard but Dad says Excessive Daytime Sleepiness is not a reason to give up your goals! He is not only the best science teacher but he is the best dad in the world, too!

Follow up questions

- What was your favorite part of the book?

- Did the book remind you of _____?

  Person in your life with Narcolepsy

- What things in the book reminded you of _____?

  Person in your life with Narcolepsy

- Does anything in the book bother you?

- Is there anything else you would like to learn about Narcolepsy and Excessive Daytime Sleepiness

Definitions

- Sleep Disorder: When a person's sleep patterns are different then they should be

- Narcolepsy: When the brain goes sleep during times the person should be awake

- Excessive Daytime Sleepiness: When a person has a hard time staying awake even after a full night's sleep.

- Symptom: When a person does something "weird" or different that lets them or others know they might be sick.

Books in the Talking to Kids About Narcolepsy Series

Book 1 - Automatic Behavior: Sometimes My Socks are in the Freezer

Book 2 - Excessive Daytime Sleepiness: My Dad Naps Too!

Coming Soon!

Book 3 - Cataplexy

Book 4 - Sleep Paralysis

Book 5 - Hypnagogic Hallucinations

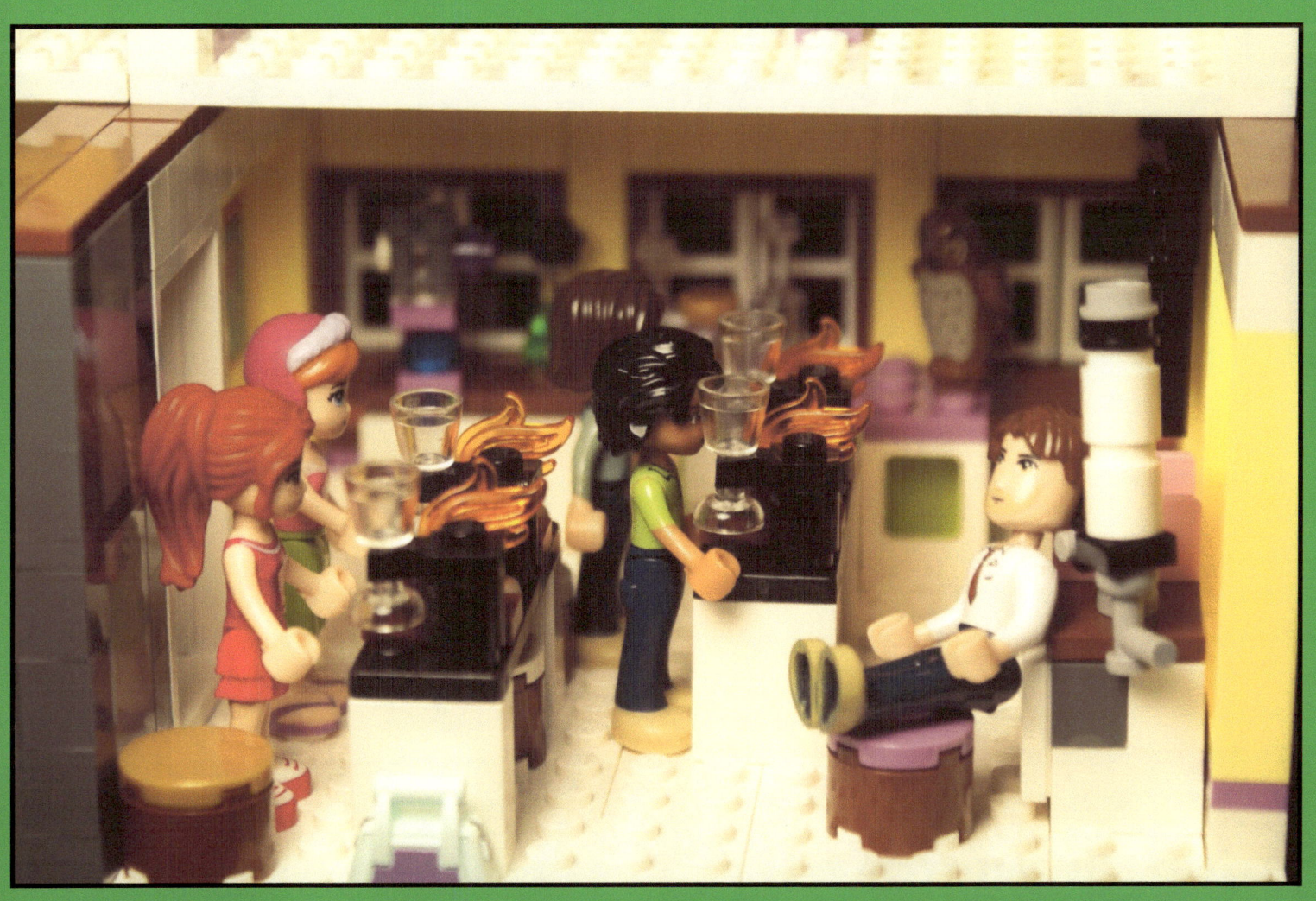

About the Author

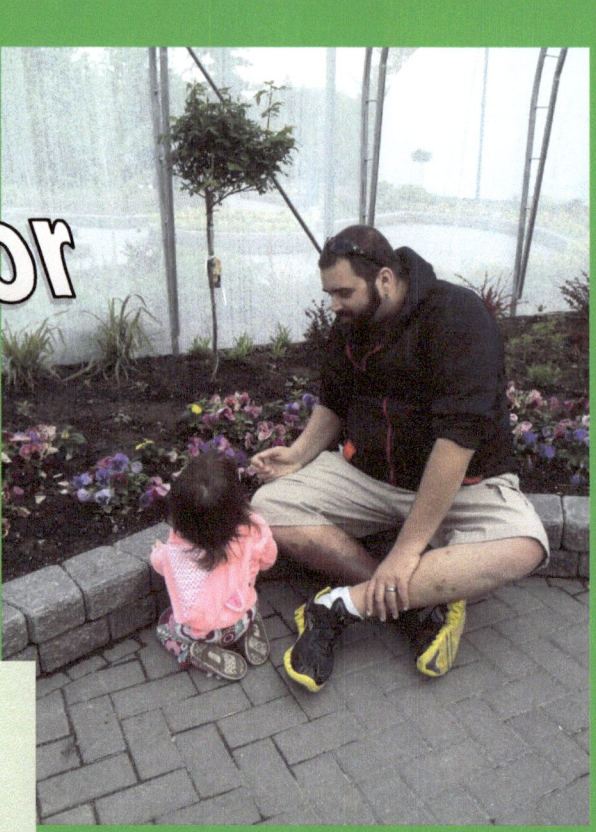

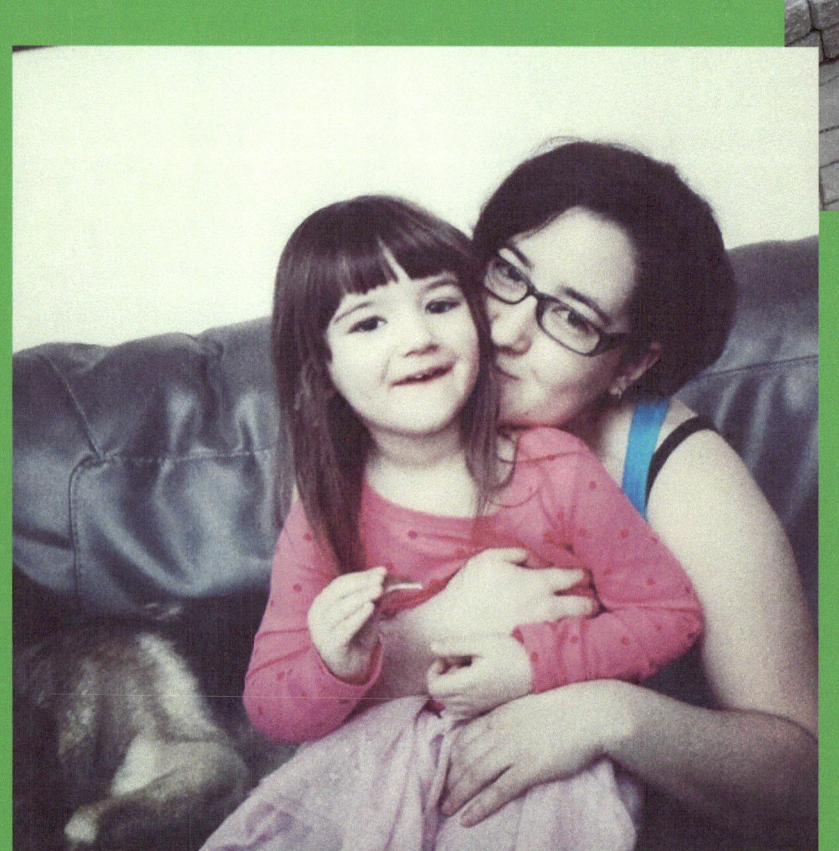

Amanda Stock is the author and photographer of My Dad Naps Too! and the upcoming books in the Talking to Kids about Narcolepsy series. These books were written to assist adults with explaining what Narcolepsy is to a young child or other people in their life. Having a young daughter, Amanda knew this would be an obstacle she would one day face and set out to find a solution.

Amanda is a wife and mother living with Narcolepsy. Like most Narcoleptics she began showing symptoms at age 15 but was not diagnosed unto age 26. Receiving that diagnosis was a huge relief. Understanding what the problem was and how to manage it has made a big difference in her life.

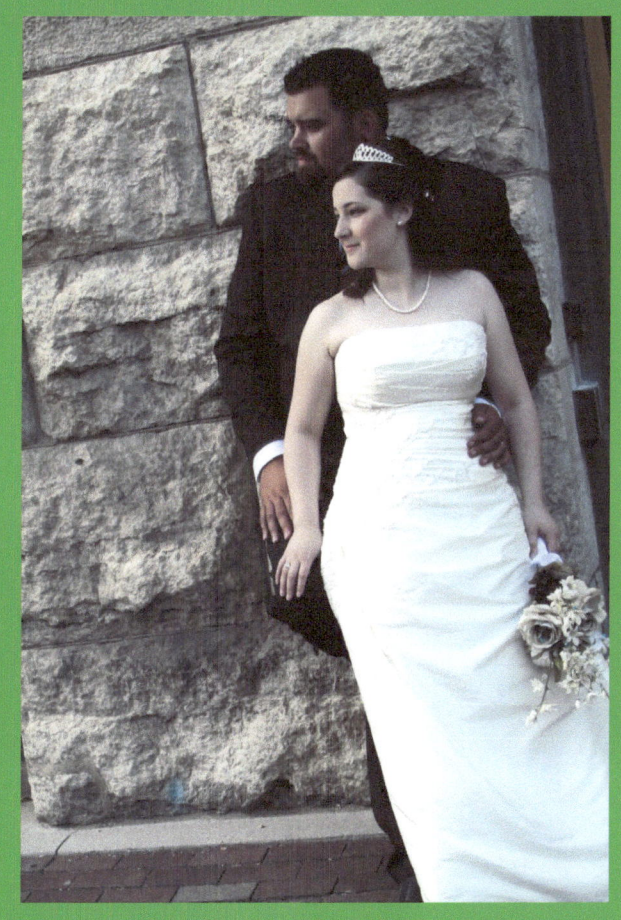

The Talking to Kids about Narcolepsy book series has been a three year project due to the author's incredible lack of drawing skills. This book series is in no way authorized, sponsored, or endorsed by The LEGO Company but could not have completed without their amazing product.

www.ingramcontent.com/pod-product-compliance
Lightning Source LLC
Chambersburg PA
CBHW060828290526
45792CB00005BB/1845